Renal diet for beginners

A comprehensive guide with healthy and delicious recipes to manage kidney disease with ease

Carol Hannigan

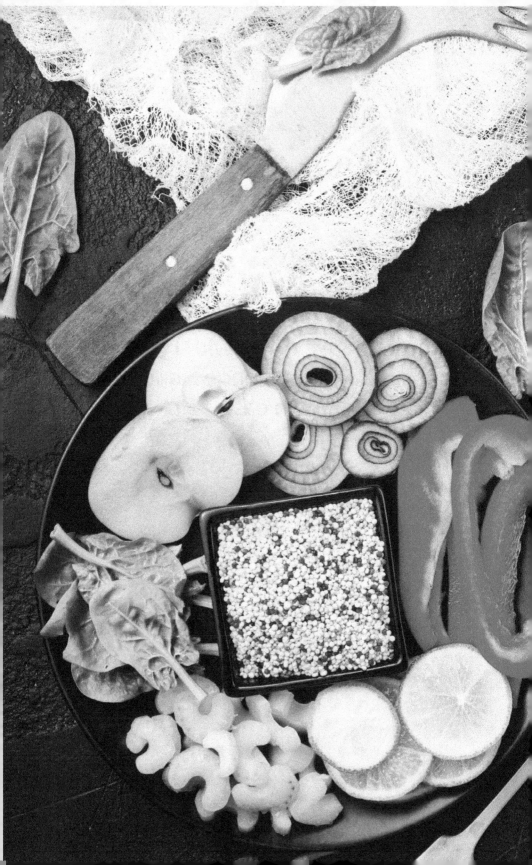

The following Book is reproduced below with the goal of providing information that is as accurate and reliable as possible. Regardless, purchasing this Book can be seen as consent to the fact that both the publisher and the author of this book are in no way experts on the topics discussed within and that any recommendations or suggestions that are made herein are for entertainment purposes only. Professionals should be consulted as needed prior to undertaking any of the action endorsed herein.

This declaration is deemed fair and valid by both the American Bar Association and the Committee of Publishers Association and is legally binding throughout the United States.

Furthermore, the transmission, duplication, or reproduction of any of the following work including specific information will be considered an illegal act irrespective of if it is done electronically or in print. This extends to creating a secondary or tertiary copy of the work or a recorded copy and is only allowed with the express written consent from the Publisher. All additional right reserved.

The information in the following pages is broadly considered a truthful and accurate account of facts and as such, any inattention, use, or misuse of the information in question by the reader will render any resulting actions solely under their purview. There are no scenarios in which the publisher or the

Table of content

Chapter 1. What is kidney disease?

Chronic kidney disease describes a clinical picture in which, due to various causes, there is a progressive loss of all the kidney functions. Chronic kidney disease is referred to as when the reduced kidney function persists for three months or more. The disease becomes more common with age: while around 3% of young and middle-aged people are affected, more than 10% of those aged 70–80 have chronic renal impairment. However, this disease is frequently not known to those affected because initially, only the urine and blood levels change, but no complaints occur.

For this reason, laboratory values play an important role in early detection as well as regular monitoring in patients at high risk of developing chronic kidney disease.

Nearly 60% of patients with chronic kidney disease have long-standing diabetes or hypertension. These groups are, therefore, the focus of regular screening for kidney damage. Important protection against chronic kidney disease is the prevention of diabetes and hypertension and their consistent treatment.

Chronic kidney disease progresses even with optimal treatment mostly slowly over months to years. Chronic kidney disease is to be differentiated from acute renal failure. Acute renal failure develops rapidly within a few days and can regress with proper therapy without causing damage. Again, different diseases can be the cause. Many patients are already in poor overall condition if they develop acute renal failure. Circulatory failure in the context of blood poisoning is an example of such a serious underlying disease.

Chapter 2. What role do the kidneys play in our body?

There are a number of other interesting facts to consider regarding your kidneys and the important role they play in your body. Have you ever wondered about their critical function, aside from ridding the body of toxins? The kidneys perform a number of tasks, which makes their ability to work well and efficiently one of the most important functions of the body. Knowing what they do and how they do it can provide you with a new level of appreciation and understanding about why it is so vital to ensure they are supported:

- Kidneys regulate water, electrolytes, and blood pressure. They pump out a significant amount of sodium and make sure our bodies are balanced to the optimum levels for optimal function and performance. When there is too much of anything, they will release it, which makes it crucial to avoid consuming excessive levels of sodium and other ingredients that can cause the kidneys to work "overtime" and eventually slow down.

- An enzyme produced by the kidneys called rennin is responsible for the regulation of sodium and blood pressure. However, to produce enough of this enzyme the kidneys must be able to function well.

- When we reduce the number of carbohydrates in our diet, either for health or weight loss goals, our kidneys help produce a form of glucose that our body needs for fuel once our own fat stores are depleted. This process occurs by using amino acids to create glucose. When this occurs, it becomes increasingly more important that our kidneys are at their optimal level. Otherwise, they are unable to produce this source of fuel, and the results can be serious—including fatal. Changing your diet should always be a personal choice, though it's best to check with a medical professional before proceeding with any diet, especially where kidney function becomes a factor.

- A lesser-known fact about kidneys is their ability to convert vitamin D into a useful nutrient in our bodies once we absorb it through sunlight or other sources. When we absorb this vitamin, it has no "active" value unless it is processed by the kidneys for its benefits. This means that even if we get the amount of vitamin D we need, it has no value until it reaches the kidneys.

The kidneys not only rid the body of waste, but they are also responsible for processing and converting nutrients into forms that can be used to support our body's health as a whole and ensure we get the most out of what we absorb and consume.

Chapter 3. kidney failure: causes and symptoms

Your kidneys are a pair of organs located toward your lower back. One kidney is on each side of your spine. They filter your blood and remove toxins from your body. Kidneys send toxins to your bladder, which your body later removes toxins during urination.

Kidney failure occurs when your kidneys lose the ability to sufficiently filter waste from your blood. Many factors can interfere with your kidney health and function, such as:

- toxic exposure to environmental pollutants or certain medications
- certain acute and chronic diseases
- severe dehydration
- kidney trauma

Your body becomes overloaded with toxins if your kidneys can't do their regular job. This can lead to kidney failure, which can be life-threatening if left untreated.

Symptoms of kidney failure

Usually someone with kidney failure will have a few symptoms of the disease. Sometimes no symptoms are present. Possible symptoms include:

- a reduced amount of urine

- swelling of your legs, ankles, and feet from retention of fluids caused by the failure of the kidneys to eliminate water waste

- unexplained shortness of breath

- excessive drowsiness or fatigue

- persistent nausea

- confusion

- pain or pressure in your chest

- seizures

Causes of kidney failure

Kidney failure can be the result of several conditions or causes. The cause typically also determines the type of kidney failure.

People who are most at risk usually have one or more of the following causes:

Loss of blood flow to the kidneys

A sudden loss of blood flow to your kidneys can prompt kidney failure. Some conditions that cause loss of blood flow to the kidneys include:

- a heart attack
- heart disease
- scarring of the liver or liver failure
- dehydration
- a severe burn
- an allergic reaction
- a severe infection, such as sepsis

High blood pressure and anti-inflammatory medications can also limit blood flow.

Chapter 4. The Benefits of Renal Diet

- **A renal diet minimizes the intake of sodium, potassium, and phosphorus.** Excessive sodium is harmful to people who have been diagnosed with kidney disease, as this causes fluid build-up, making it hard for the kidneys to eliminate sodium and fluid.

- **Improper functioning of the kidneys can also mean difficulty in removing excess potassium.** When there is too much potassium in the body, this can lead to a condition called hyperkalaemia, which can also cause problems with the heart and blood vessels.

- **Kidneys that are not working efficiently have difficulty removing excess phosphorus.** High levels of phosphorus excrete calcium from the bones causing them to weaken. This also causes elevation of calcium deposits in the eyes, heart, lungs, and blood vessels.

Table with the Nutritional Values of Foods

- A renal diet focuses on foods that are natural and nutritious, but at the same time, are low in sodium, potassium, and phosphorus.
- Foods to Eat
- **Cauliflower** – 1 cup contains 19 mg sodium, 176 potassium, 40 mg phosphorus.
- **Blueberries** – 1 cup contains 1.5 mg sodium, 114 potassium, 18 mg phosphorus.
- **Sea Bass** – 3 ounces contain 74 mg sodium, 279 potassium, 211 mg phosphorus.
- **Grapes** – 1/2 cup contains 1.5 mg sodium, 144 potassium, 15 mg phosphorus.
- **Egg Whites** – 2 egg whites contain 110 mg sodium, 108 potassium, 10 mg phosphorus.
- **Garlic** – 3 cloves contain 1.5 mg sodium, 36 potassium, 14 mg phosphorus.
- **Buckwheat** – ½ cup contains 3.5 mg sodium, 74 potassium, 59 mg phosphorus.
- **Olive Oil** – 1 ounce 0.6 mg sodium, 0.3 potassium, 0 mg phosphorus.
- **Bulgur** – ½ cup contains 4.5 mg sodium, 62 potassium, 36 mg phosphorus.

- **Cabbage** – 1 cup contains 13 mg sodium, 119 potassium, 18 mg phosphorus.
- **Skinless chicken** – 3 ounces contain 63 mg sodium, 216 potassium, 192 mg phosphorus.
- **Bell peppers** – 1 piece contains 3 mg sodium, 156 potassium, 19 mg phosphorus.
- **Onion** – 1 piece contains 3 mg sodium, 102 potassium, 20 mg phosphorus.
- **Arugula** – 1 cup contains 6 mg sodium, 74 potassium, 10 mg phosphorus.
- **Macadamia nuts** – 1 ounce contains 1.4 mg sodium, 103 potassium, 53 mg phosphorus.
- **Radish** – ½ cup contains 23 mg sodium, 135 potassium, 12 mg phosphorus.
- **Turnips** – ½ cup contains 12.5 mg sodium, 138 potassium, 20 mg phosphorus.
- **Pineapple** – 1 cup contains 2 mg sodium, 180 potassium, 13 mg phosphorus.
- **Cranberries** – 1 cup contains 2 mg sodium, 85 potassium, 13 mg phosphorus.
- **Mushrooms** – 1 cup contains 6 mg sodium, 170 potassium, 42 mg phosphorus.

Foods to Avoid

These foods are known to have high levels of potassium, sodium or phosphorus:

- **Soda** – Soda is believed to contain up to 100 mg of additive phosphorus per 200 ml.

- **Avocados** – 1 cup contains up to 727 mg of potassium.

- **Canned foods** – Canned foods contain high amounts of sodium so make sure that you avoid using these, or at least, opt for low-sodium versions.

- **Whole wheat bread** – 1 ounce of bread contains 57 mg phosphorus and 69 mg potassium, which is higher compared to white bread.

- **Brown rice** – 1 cup of brown rice contains 154 mg potassium, while 1 cup of white rice only has 54 mg potassium.

- **Bananas** – 1 banana contains 422 mg of potassium.

- **Dairy** – Dairy products are high in potassium, phosphorus, and calcium. You can still consume dairy products, but you have to limit it. Use dairy milk alternatives like almond milk and coconut milk.

- **Processed meats** – Processed meats are not advisable for people with kidney problems because of their high content of additives and preservatives.

- **Pickled and cured foods** – These are made using large amounts of salt.

- **Apricots** – 1 cup contains 427 mg potassium.

- **Potatoes and sweet potatoes** – 1 potato contain 610 mg potassium. You can double boil potatoes and sweet potatoes to reduce potassium by 50 percent.

- **Tomatoes** – 1 cup tomato sauce contains up to 900 mg potassium.

- **Instant meals** – Instant meals are known for extremely high amounts of sodium.

- **Raisins, prunes, and dates –** Dried fruits have concentrated nutrients, including potassium. 1 cup of prunes contain up to 1,274 mg potassium.

Breakfast

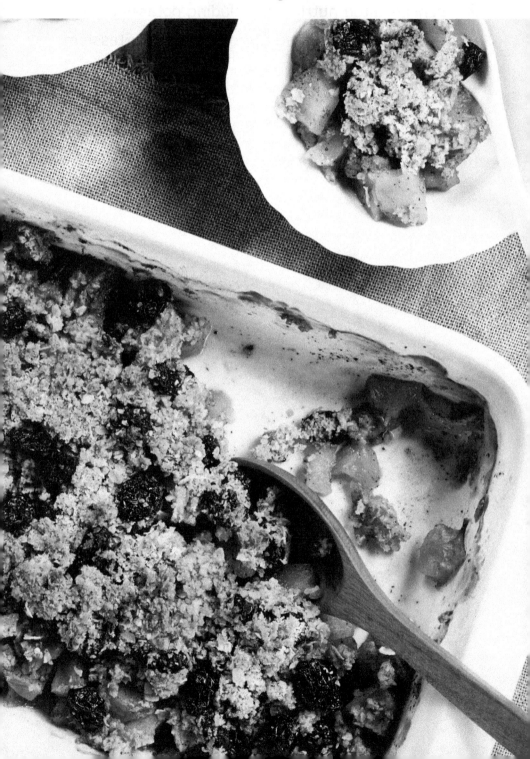

1. Healthy Egg White and Broccoli Omelette

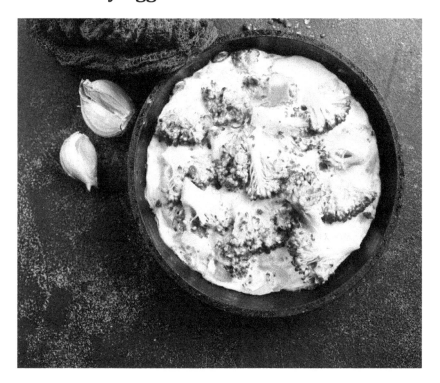

Preparation time: 10 minutes.

Cooking time: 20 minutes.

Servings: 2

Ingredients

- 2 large egg whites
- 1 teaspoon olive oil
- Dash of black pepper
- Dash of oregano

- 3 tablespoons chopped broccoli

- 1 tablespoon whole milk

Direction

- Separate the yolk from the egg whites in two large eggs, placing the whites in a medium-sized bowl. Mix black pepper, oregano, broccoli, and milk. The amount of froth equals how fluffy your omelet will be.

- Put the olive oil on the frying pan and let heat for about a minute before adding the egg mixture. Let sit until the liquid becomes solid, and then flip for about a minute.

- Enjoy!

Nutrition

Calories: 90.3kcal

Total fat: 5.1g

Saturated fat: 0g

Cholesterol: 1.2mg

Sodium: 122.4mg

Total carbs: 2.1g

Fiber: 0.9g

Sugar: 0g

Protein: 9.1g

2. Breakfast Casserole

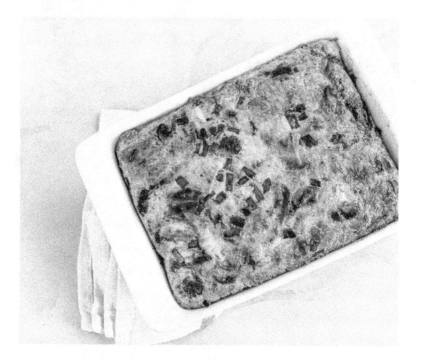

Preparation Time: 10 minutes

Cooking Time: 60 minutes

Servings: 8

Ingredients

- 200 grams of ground lean beef – fresh and grass-fed if possible
- ½ cup cream cheese
- 4 slices of bread – white, cut in cubes
- 5 eggs
- 1 teaspoon of mustard – dry
- ½ teaspoon garlic powder with no added sodium

Direction:

- Preheat your oven to 350 degrees F as you are preparing ingredients for breakfast casserole. Cube bread sliced and place it aside while you are taking care of the ground beef.
- As you prepare the beef, add a tablespoon of olive oil to the skillet and add the beef. Cook the beef with occasional stirring as you are breaking the meat parts to bits. Once the meat is browned, set aside and add garlic powder, stirring it well to combine.
- Beat the five eggs in a bowl then combine all ingredients in the egg bowl, mixing to get a homogenous mass out of the egg mixture. Pour the mixture into the mildly greased baking dish and place it in the oven. Bake for 50 minutes or until ready.

Nutrition:

Potassium 176 mg

Sodium 201 mg

Phosphorus 119 mg

Calories 220

3. Grilled Veggie and Cheese Bagel

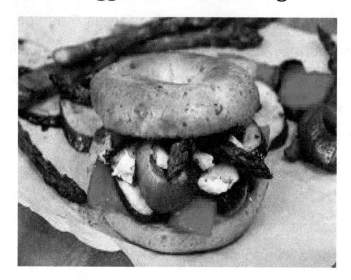

Preparation time: 10 minutes.

Cooking time: 5 minutes.

Servings: 1

Ingredients

- 1 white flour bagel, sliced in half

- ½ cup arugula

- ½ cup low-sodium cheese or cream cheese (lower potassium, higher sodium)

- ¼ red onion, finely sliced

- 2 slices eggplant, roasted or grilled

- ½ teaspoon lemon pepper

Direction

- First, you need to prepare veggies and slice them, and once the preparation is finished, grill 2 slices of eggplant with some lemon pepper spread over the slices.

- Baking the eggplant slices would be another option in case you don't have an option to grill the slices. You may roast the eggplant by placing it on a tin foil or a baking paper set on a baking dish in a preheated oven for 5 minutes each side of the slices.

- Once the eggplant is grilled, toast the bagel sliced in two to make a sandwich the same way the eggplant was grilled, but reduced to grilling each side 2 minutes or less.

- Spread some cheese on the bagel, add the eggplant slices and the rest of the ingredients. Seal the bagel with the top part and you will have a great start to the day.

Nutrition

Potassium: 112mg

Sodium: 186mg

Phosphorus: 50mg

Calories: 114kcal

4. Cauliflower Tortilla

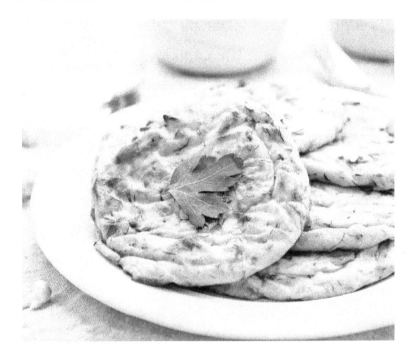

Preparation Time: 10 minutes

Cooking Time: 20 minutes

Servings: 4

Ingredients

- 4 cups cauliflower
- 1 cup onion – chopped
- 2 garlic cloves – minced
- 1 cup egg substitute - liquefied
- ¼ teaspoon nutmeg
- 1 tablespoon parsley – fresh, chopped
- ½ teaspoon allspice

Direction:

- Prepare the cauliflower by cutting it into small cubes, then place the cauliflower bits in a bowl with a tablespoon of water and microwave it for 5 minutes until cauliflower is crisped.
- While you are waiting for the cauliflower bits to get ready in the microwave, you may start with preparing the onion. Sauté chopped onions with 2 tablespoons of olive oil until browned, which should take around 5 minutes, then add garlic, nutmeg and allspice to the pan.
- Stir in and cook for another 1 to 2 minutes then add the cauliflower and egg substitute. Stir in all ingredients to combine the mixture then seal the pan and lower the heat.
- Cook for another 10 to 15 minutes, until cauliflower tortilla is browned. Serve by slicing the tortilla into 4 pieces.

Nutrition:

Potassium 272 mg

Sodium 148 mg

Phosphorus 78 mg

Calories 102

5. Eggs Benedict

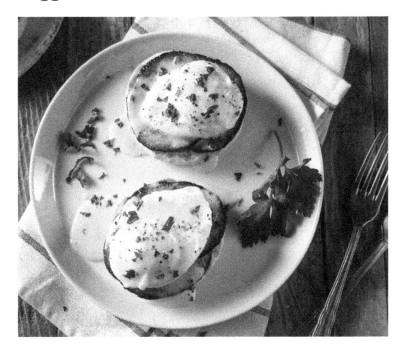

Preparation time: 10 minutes.

Cooking time: 15 minutes.

Servings: 4

Ingredients

- 2 pieces toasted bread, white flour
- 4 eggs
- 3 egg yolks
- 1 tablespoon lemon juice
- ½ teaspoon cayenne pepper
- ½ teaspoon paprika
- 1 tablespoon apple cider vinegar
- 2 tablespoons unsalted butter

Direction

- Slice the two toasted bread pieces in two, so you can end up with four pieces where each piece represents one serving.

- Take a large skillet or a pot and pour one cup of water in it. Add a tablespoon of vinegar and bring the water to boil.

- When the water starts to boil, break four eggs, one at a time, and poach the eggs by covering the skillet. Eggs should be done between 3 and 5 minutes of poaching, depending on how you like your eggs cooked.

- Next, place poached eggs on top of bread pieces. Take a skillet and add the butter so you could melt it, then add cayenne and paprika to the melted butter. Beat the egg yolks over medium heat, then add the eggs to the mixture with butter. Add lemon juice and whisk it into the egg and butter mixture.

- Once the sauce reaches an adequate thickness, remove from the heat and pour over the eggs and toasted bread.

Nutrition

Potassium: 146mg

Sodium: 206mg

Phosphorus: 114mg

Calories: 316kcal

6. Cranberry and Apple Oatmeal

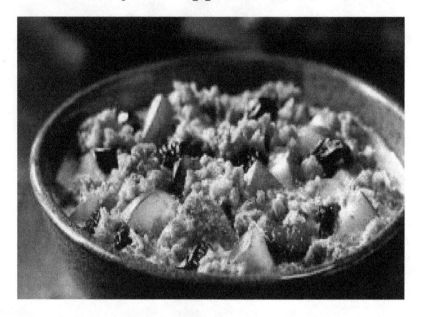

Preparation time: 10 minutes.

Cooking time: 5 minutes.

Servings: 2

Ingredients

- 1 apple, diced
- ¼ teaspoon nutmeg
- ¼ cup cranberry, fresh
- 2/3 cup oatmeal, you can use quick oatmeal with no added sodium and extra potassium; avoid whole grain if not on dialysis
- ½ teaspoon cinnamon
- 2 cup water

Direction

- First, you need to prepare all the ingredients and cut the apple into small pieces.

- Pour two cups of water into a saucepan and add the diced apple, cranberries, nutmeg, and cinnamon. Seal the saucepan and bring the water with ingredients to boil.

- Cook until the fruit is tender, which shouldn't take more than 5 to 10 minutes. Check if apples are tender, then add 2/3 cup oatmeal to the boiling water. Stir in and cook for around one minute before serving the oatmeal.

- Based on your doctor's recommendations, you can serve the oatmeal with an adequate dose of milk or add milk substitute to the oatmeal when serving.

Nutrition

Potassium: 170mg

Sodium: 59mg

Phosphorus: 187mg

Calories: 173kcal

7. Blueberry Breakfast Smoothie

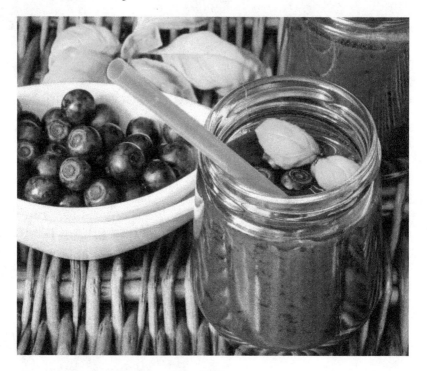

Preparation time: 5 minutes.

Cooking time: 5 minutes.

Servings: 1

Ingredients

- 1/3 cup vanilla almond milk, no sugar added

- 2 tablespoons protein powder of your choice

- ¼ cup Greek yogurt, look for brands with low sodium and low potassium

- 3 strawberries, fresh, sliced

- 6 raspberries

- 1 cup blueberries, frozen or fresh

- 1 tablespoon cereal, avoid whole grain due to high levels of potassium

Direction

- First, you need to blend one cup of blueberries in a food processor, blending the fruit at low speed for around a minute.

- After a minute, add almond milk, protein powder, and Greek yogurt to blended blueberries and blend the mixture for another minute or until the blueberry smoothie turns into a homogeneous mass.

- Pour the smoothie into a bowl, add cereals, raspberries, sliced strawberries, and serve.

Nutrition

Potassium: 270mg

Sodium: 108mg

Phosphorus: 114mg

Calories: 225kcal

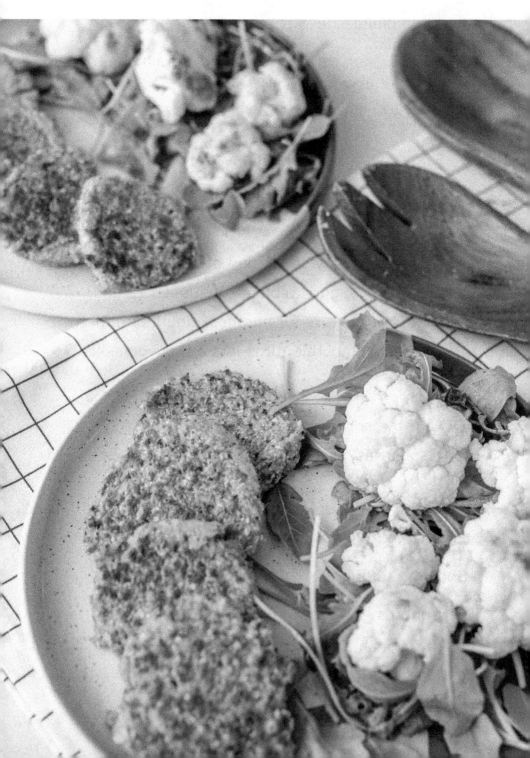

8. Tofu Stir-Fry

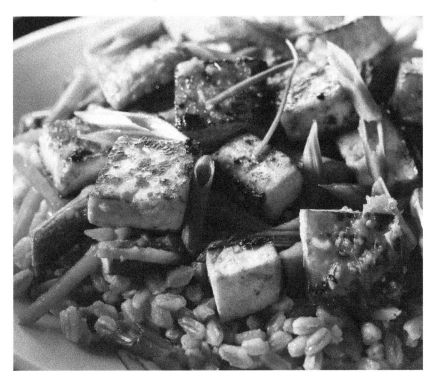

Preparation time: 20 minutes.

Cooking time: 20 minutes.

Servings: 4

Ingredients

For the tofu:

- 1 tablespoon lemon juice

- 1 teaspoon minced garlic

- 1 teaspoon grated fresh ginger

- Pinch red pepper flakes

- 5 ounces extra-firm tofu, pressed well and cubed

For the stir-fry:

- 1 tablespoon olive oil

- ½ cup cauliflower florets

- ½ cup thinly sliced carrots

- ½ cup julienned red pepper

- ½ cup fresh green beans

- 2 cup cooked white rice

Direction

- In a bowl, mix the lemon juice, garlic, ginger, and red pepper flakes.

- Add the tofu and toss to coat.

- Place the bowl in the refrigerator and marinate for 2 hours.

- To make the stir-fry, heat the oil in a skillet.

- Sauté the tofu for 8 minutes or until it is lightly browned and fully heated.

- Add the carrots and cauliflower and sauté for 5 minutes. Stirring and tossing constantly.

- Add the red pepper and green beans, sauté for 3 minutes more.

- Serve over white rice.

Nutrition

Calories: 190kcal

Fat: 6g

Carb: 30g

Phosphorus: 90mg

Potassium: 199mg

Sodium: 22mg

Protein: 6g

9. Lasagna

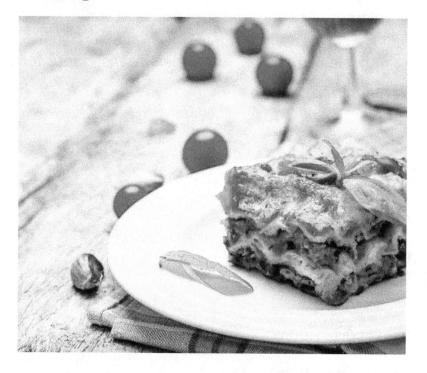

Preparation time: 10 minutes.

Cooking time: 1 hour.

Servings: 2

Ingredients

- ½ pack soft tofu

- ½ cup baby spinach

- 4 tablespoons unenriched rick milk

- 1 clove garlic, crushed

- 1 lemon, juiced

- 2 tablespoons fresh basil, chopped

- A pinch of black pepper to taste

- 1 zucchini, sliced

- 1 red bell pepper, sliced

- 1 eggplant, sliced

Direction

- Preheat the oven to 325ºF. Soak vegetables in warm water before cooking.

- In a blender, process the tofu, garlic, milk, basil, lemon juice, and pepper until smooth.

- Toss in the zucchini and spinach for the last 30 seconds.

- Layer the bottom of the dish with 1/3 eggplant slices and 1/3 red pepper slices and then cover with 1/3 of the tofu sauce. Repeat to complete.

- Bake in the oven for 1 hour or until the vegetables are soft through to the center.

- Finish under the broiler until golden and bubbly.

- Divide into portions and serve with a sprinkle of black pepper to taste.

Nutrition

Calories: 116kcal

Fat: 4g

Carb: 10g

Phosphorus: 149mg

Potassium: 346mg

Sodium: 27mg

Protein: 5g

10. Cauliflower Patties

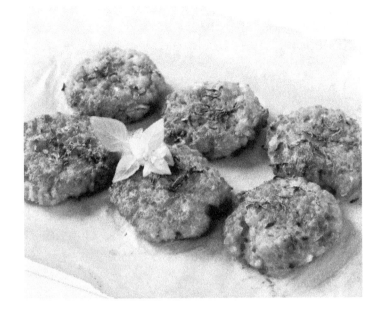

Preparation time: 5 minutes.

Cooking time: 8 minutes.

Servings: 2

Ingredients

- 2 eggs
- 2 egg whites
- ½ onion, diced
- 2 cups cauliflower, frozen
- 2 tablespoons all-purpose white flour
- 1 teaspoon black pepper

- 1 tablespoon coconut oil

- 1 teaspoon curry powder

- 1 tablespoon fresh cilantro

Direction:

- Soak vegetables in warm water before cooking.

- Steam cauliflower over a pan of boiling water for 10 minutes.

- Blend eggs and onion in a food processor before adding cooked cauliflower, spices, cilantro, flour, and pepper and blast in the processor for 30 seconds.

- Heat a skillet on high heat and add oil.

- Pour tablespoons portions of the cauliflower mixture into the pan and brown on each side until crispy, about 3 to 4 minutes.

- Enjoy with a salad.

Nutrition

Calories: 227kcal

Fat: 12g

Carb: 15g

Phosphorus: 193mg

Potassium: 513mg

Sodium: 158mg

Protein: 13g

11. Turnip Chips

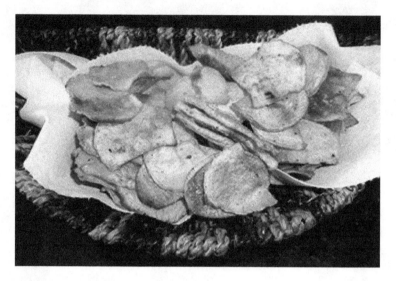

Preparation time: 5 minutes.

Cooking time: 50 minutes.

Servings: 2

Ingredients

- 2 turnips, peeled and sliced

- 1 tablespoon extra-virgin olive oil

- 1 onion, chopped

- 1 clove minced garlic

- 1 teaspoon black pepper

- 1 teaspoon oregano

- 1 teaspoon paprika

Direction

- Preheat oven to 375ºF. Grease a baking tray with olive oil.

- Add turnip slices in a thin layer.

- Dust over herbs and spices with an extra drizzle of olive oil.

- Bake 40 minutes. Turning once.

Nutrition

Calories: 136kcal

Fat: 14g

Carb: 30g

Phosphorus: 50mg

Potassium: 356mg

Sodium: 71mg

Protein: 0g

12. Mock Pancakes

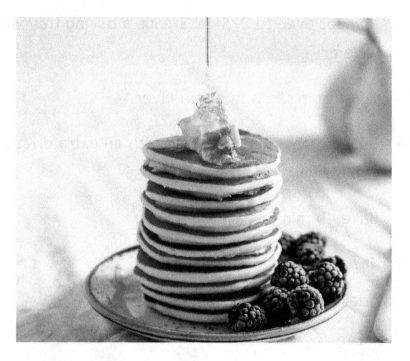

Preparation time: 5 minutes.

Cooking time: 5 minutes.

Servings: 2

Ingredients

- 2 tablespoons honey

- 1 teaspoon cinnamon

- 1 cup ricotta cheese

- 1 egg

Directions

- Using a blender, put together egg, honey, cinnamon, and ricotta cheese. Process until all ingredients are well combined.

- Pour an equal amount of the blended mixture into the pan. Cook each pancake for 4 minutes on both sides. Serve.

Nutrition

Calories: 188.1kcal

Protein: 16.84g

Potassium (K): 177mg

Sodium (Na): 136mg

Fat: 14.5 g

Carbs: 5.5g

Phosphorus: 134mg

Meat and Poultry

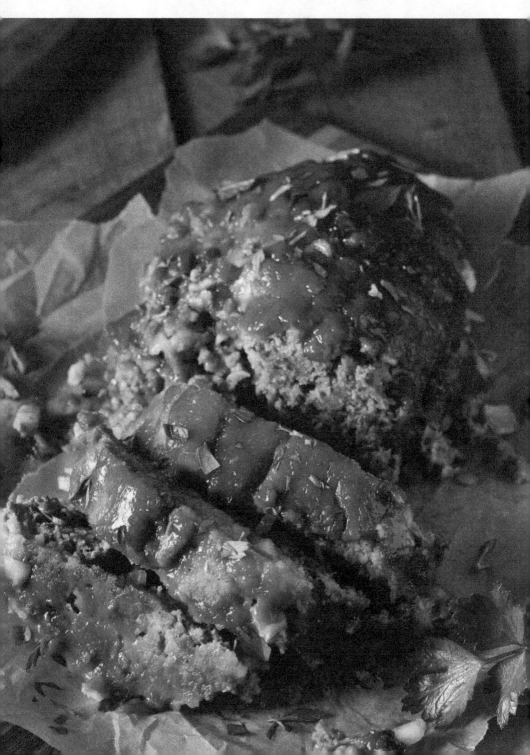

13. Country Fried Steak

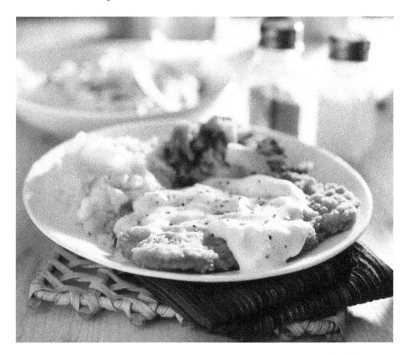

Preparation time: 10 minutes.

Cooking time: 100 minutes.

Servings: 3

Ingredients

- 1 large onion

- ½ cup flour

- 3 tablespoons vegetable oil

- ¼ teaspoon pepper

- 1½ pounds round steak

- ½ teaspoon paprika

Direction

- Trim excess fat from steak

- Cut into small pieces

- Combine flour, paprika, and pepper and mix.

- Preheat skillet with oil

- Cook steak on both sides

- When the color of steak is brown, remove to a platter

- Add water (150 ml) and stir around the skillet

- Return browned steak to skillet; if necessary, add water again so that the bottom side of steak does not stick

Nutrition

Calories: 248kcal

Protein: 30g

Fat: 10g

Carbs: 5g

Phosphorus: 190mg

Potassium (K): 338mg

Sodium (Na): 60mg

14. Beef Pot Roast

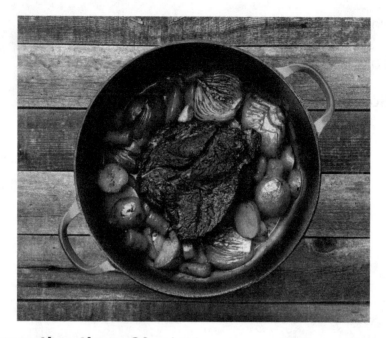

Preparation time: 20 minutes

Cooking time: 60 minutes

Servings: 3

Ingredients:

- Round bone roast
- 2 - 4 lbs. chuck roast

Direction:

- Trim off excess fat
- Place a tablespoon of oil in a large skillet and heat to medium

- Roll pot roast in flour and brown on all sides in a hot skillet
- After the meat gets a brown color, reduce heat to low
- Season with pepper and herbs and add ½ cup of water
- Cook slowly for 1½ hours or until it looks ready

Nutrition:

Calories 157,

Protein 24 g,

Fat 13 g,

Carbs 0 g,

Phosphorus 204 mg,

Potassium (K) 328 mg,

Sodium (Na) 50 mg

15. Meat Loaf

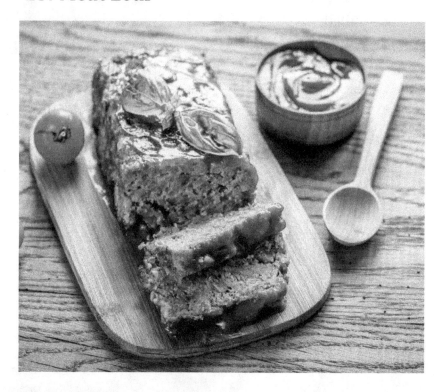

Preparation time: 20 minutes.

Cooking time: 20 minutes.

Servings: 1

Ingredients

- ½ teaspoon ground sage
- 1 egg
- ¼ teaspoon garlic powder
- 1 cup milk
- 1 tablespoon chopped parsley

- 4 soft bread slices

- ½ pound lean ground pork

- ¼ teaspoon pepper

- ¼ teaspoon mustard

- 1 pound lean ground beef

- ¼ cup onion

Direction

- Heat oven at 350°F.

- Mix elements in a bowl.

- Place mixture in a shallow baking dish.

- Bake ½ hours or until done (At the end, the loaf should be crispy brown).

Nutrition

Calories: 261kcal

Protein: 27g

Fat: 12g

Carbs: 8g

Phosphorus: 244mg

Potassium (K): 450mg

Sodium (Na): 180mg

16. Spiced Lamb Burgers

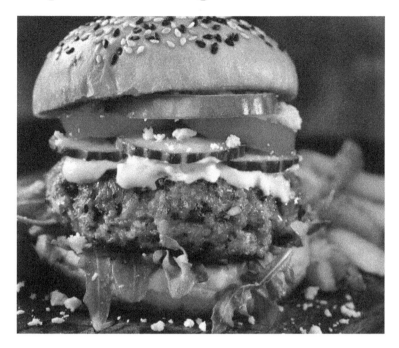

Preparation time: 10 minutes.

Cooking time: 20 minutes.

Servings: 2

Ingredients

- 1 tablespoon extra-virgin olive oil

- 1 teaspoon cumin

- ½ finely diced red onion

- 1 minced garlic clove

- 1 teaspoon harissa spices

- 1 cup arugula

- 1 juiced lemon

- 6-ounces lean ground lamb

- 1 tablespoon parsley

- ½ cup low-fat plain yogurt

Direction

- Preheat the broiler on medium to high heat.

- Mix the ground lamb, red onion, parsley, Harissa spices, and olive oil until combined.

- Shape 1-inch thick patties using wet hands.

- Add the patties to a baking tray and place them under the broiler for 7–8 minutes on each side or until well cooked

- Mix the yogurt, lemon juice, and cumin and serve over the lamb burgers with a side salad of arugula.

Nutrition

Calories: 306kcal

Fat: 20g

Carbs: 10g

Phosphorus: 269mg

Potassium (K): 492mg

Sodium (Na): 86mg

Protein: 23g

17. Pork Loins with Leeks

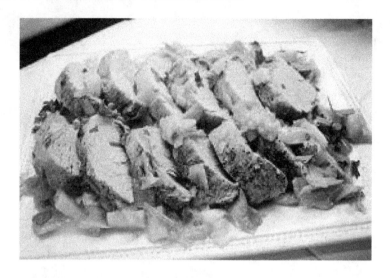

Preparation time: 10 minutes.

Cooking time: 35 minutes.

Servings: 2

Ingredients

- 1 sliced leek
- 1 tablespoon mustard seeds
- 6-ounces pork tenderloin
- 1 tablespoon cumin seeds
- 1 tablespoon dry mustard
- 1 tablespoon extra-virgin oil

Direction

- Preheat the broiler to medium-high heat.

- In a dry skillet, heat mustard and cumin seeds until they start to pop (3–5 minutes).

- Grind seeds using a pestle and mortar or blender and then mix in the dry mustard.

- Coat the pork on both sides with the mustard blend and add to a baking tray to broil for 25–30 minutes or until well cooked. Turn once halfway through.

- Remove and place to one side.

- Heat the oil in a pan on medium heat and add the leeks for 5–6 minutes or until soft.

- Serve the pork tenderloin on a bed of leeks and enjoy it!

Nutrition

Calories: 139kcal

Fat: 5g

Carbs: 2g

Phosphorus: 278mg

Potassium (K): 45mg

Sodium (Na): 47mg

Protein :18g

Fish and seafood

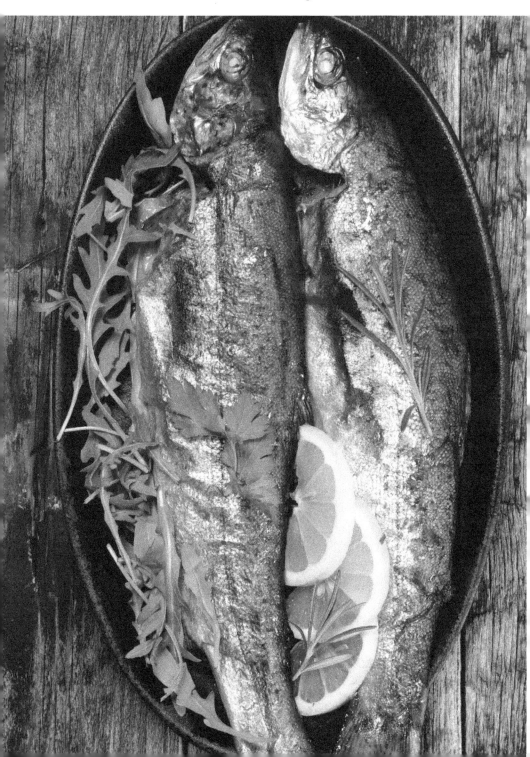

18. Shrimp Paella

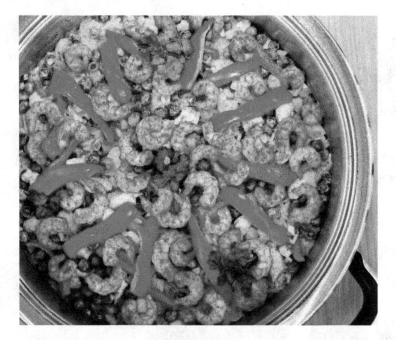

Preparation time: 5 minutes.

Cooking time: 10 minutes.

Servings: 2

Ingredients

- 1 cup cooked brown rice

- 1 chopped red onion

- 1 teaspoon paprika

- 1 chopped garlic clove

- 1 tablespoon olive oil

- 6-ounces frozen cooked shrimp

- 1 deseeded and sliced chili pepper

- 1 tablespoon oregano

Direction

- Heat the olive oil in a large pan on medium-high heat.

- Add the onion and garlic and sauté for 2–3 minutes until soft.

- Now add the shrimp and sauté for a further 5 minutes or until very hot.

- Now add the herbs, spices, chili, and rice with 1/2 cup boiling water.

- Stir until everything is warm and the water has been absorbed.

- Plate up and serve.

Nutrition

Calories: 221kcal

Protein: 17g

Carbs: 31g

Fat: 8g

Sodium (Na): 235mg

Potassium (K): 176mg

Phosphorus: 189mg

19. Grilled Salmon

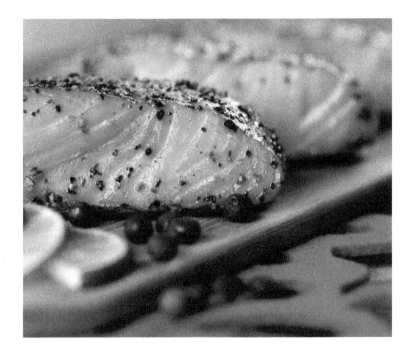

Preparation time: 15 minutes.

Cooking time: 15 minutes.

Servings: 4

Ingredients

- 1 pound salmon fillets
- 1 tablespoon olive oil
- 1 teaspoon salt-free lemon pepper
- 1/2 teaspoon paprika

Directions

- Preheat grill on high heat.

- Spray or brush fillet side of the salmon fillets lightly with oil. Combine seasonings in a small bowl. Sprinkle evenly over fillets.

- Place salmon directly on the grill, fillet side down; cook for 4 minutes. Spray or brush skin lightly with oil. Turn fillets over and cook until fish flakes easily with a fork, about 3 to 5 minutes.

Nutrition

Calories: 114kcal

Sodium: 22mg

Protein: 11.9g

Potassium: 80mg

Phosphorus: 67mg

20. Salmon Stuffed Pasta

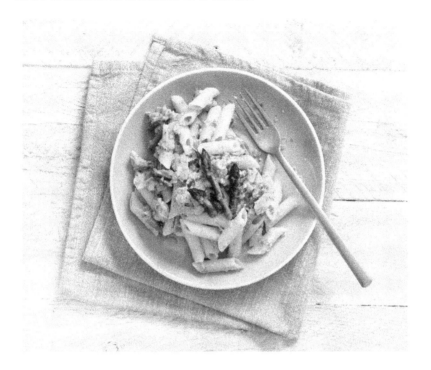

Preparation time: 10 minutes.

Cooking time: 35 minutes.

Servings: 24

Ingredients

- 24 jumbo pasta shells, boiled

- 1 cup coffee creamer

Filling:

- 2 eggs, beaten

- 2 cups creamed cottage cheese

- ¼ cup chopped onion

- 1 red bell pepper, diced

- 2 teaspoons dried parsley

- ½ teaspoon lemon peel

- 1 can salmon, drained

Dill Sauce:

- 1 ½ teaspoon butter

- 1 ½ teaspoon flour

- 1/8 teaspoon pepper

- 1 tablespoon lemon juice

- 1 ½ cup coffee creamer

- 2 teaspoons dried dill weed

Directions

- Beat the egg with the cream cheese and all the other filling ingredients in a bowl.

- Divide the filling in the pasta shells and place the shells in a 9x13 baking dish.

- Pour the coffee creamer around the stuffed shells, then cover with a foil.

- Bake the shells for 30 minutes at 350ºF.

- Meanwhile, whisk all the ingredients for dill sauce in a saucepan.

- Stir for 5 minutes until it thickens.

- Pour this sauce over the baked pasta shells.

- Serve warm.

Nutrition

Calories: 268

Total fat: 4.8g

Saturated fat: 2g

Cholesterol: 27mg

Sodium: 86mg

Total carbohydrate: 42.6g

Phosphorous: 314mg

Potassium: 181mg

21. Herbed Vegetable Trout

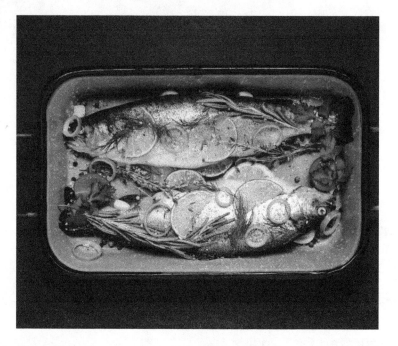

Preparation time: 10 minutes.

Cooking time: 15 minutes.

Servings: 4

Ingredients

- 14-ounces trout fillets

- 1/2 teaspoon herb seasoning blend

- 1 lemon, sliced

- 2 green onions, sliced

- 1 stalk celery, chopped

- 1 medium carrot, julienne

Directions

- Prepare and preheat a charcoal grill over moderate heat.

- Place the trout fillets over a large piece of foil and drizzle herb seasoning on top.

- Spread the lemon slices, carrots, celery, and green onions over the fish.

- Cover the fish with foil and pack it.

- Place the packed fish in the grill and cook for 15 minutes.

- Once done, remove the foil from the fish.

- Serve.

Nutrition

Calories: 202kcal

Total Fat: 8.5g

Saturated Fat: 1.5g

Cholesterol: 73mg

Sodium: 82mg

Carbohydrate: 3.5g

Phosphorous: 287mg

Potassium: 560mg

22. Citrus Glazed Salmon

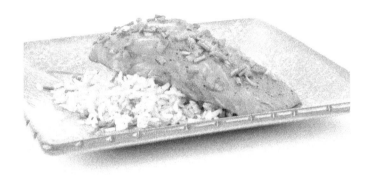

Preparation time: 10 minutes.

Cooking time: 17 minutes.

Servings: 2

Ingredients

- 2 garlic cloves, crushed

- 1 1/2 tablespoons lemon juice

- 2 tablespoons olive oil

- 1 tablespoon butter

- 1 tablespoon Dijon mustard

- 2 dashes cayenne pepper

- 1 teaspoon dried basil leaves

- 1 teaspoon dried dill

- 24-ounces salmon filet

Directions

- Place a 1-quart saucepan over moderate heat and add the oil, butter, garlic, lemon juice, mustard, cayenne pepper, dill, and basil to the pan.

- Stir this mixture for 5 minutes after it has boiled.

- Prepare and preheat a charcoal grill over moderate heat.

- Place the fish on a foil sheet and fold the edges to make a foil tray.

- Pour the prepared sauce over the fish.

- Place the fish in the foil in the preheated grill and cook for 12 minutes.

- Slice and serve.

Nutrition

Calories: 401

Total fat: 20.5g

Saturated fat: 5.3g

Cholesterol: 144mg

Sodium: 256mg

Carbohydrate: 0.5g

Phosphorous: 214mg

Potassium: 446mg

Soups

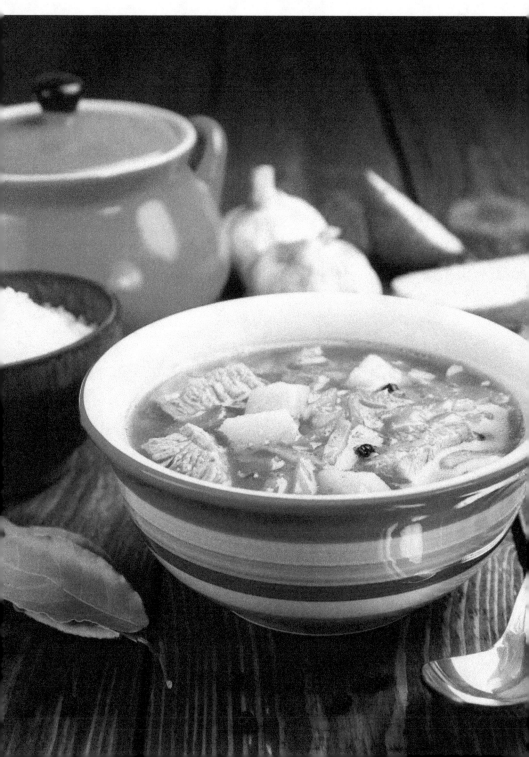

23. Classic Chicken Soup

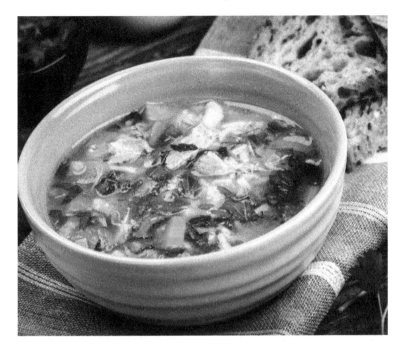

Preparation time: 10 minutes.

Cooking time: 35 minutes.

Servings: 2

Ingredients

- 2 teaspoons minced garlic
- 2 celery stalks, chopped
- 1 tablespoon unsalted butter
- ½ sweet onion, diced
- 1 carrot, diced

- 4 cups of water

- 1 teaspoon chopped fresh thyme

- 2 cups chopped cooked chicken breast

- 1 cup chicken stock

- Black pepper (ground), to taste

- 2 tablespoons chopped fresh parsley

Directions

- Take a medium-large cooking pot, heat oil over medium heat.

- Add onion and stir-cook until become translucent and softened.

- Add garlic and stir-cook until you become fragrant.

- Add celery, carrot, chicken, chicken stock, and water.

- Boil the mixture.

- Over low heat, simmer the mixture for about 25–30 minutes until veggies are tender.

- Mix in thyme and cook for 2 minutes; season to taste with black pepper.

- Serve warm with parsley on top.

Nutrition

Calories: 135kcal

Fat: 6g

Phosphorus: 122mg

Potassium: 208mg

Sodium: 74mg

Carbohydrates: 3g

Protein: 15g

24. Beef Okra Soup

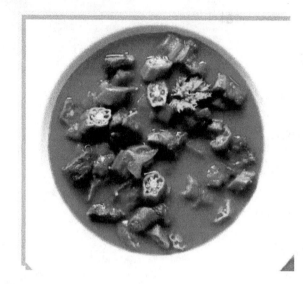

Preparation time: 10 minutes.

Cooking time: 45 minutes.

Servings: 5

Ingredients

- ½ cup okra
- ½ teaspoon basil
- ½ cup carrots, diced
- 3 ½ cups water
- 1 pound beef stew meat
- 1 cup raw sliced onions
- ½ cup green peas

- 1 teaspoon black pepper

- ½ teaspoon thyme

- ½ cup corn kernels

Directions

- Take a medium-large cooking pot, heat oil over medium heat.

- Add water, beef stew meat, black pepper, onions, basil, thyme, and stir-cook for 40–45 minutes until meat is tender.

- Add all veggies. Over low heat, simmer the mixture for about 20–25 minutes. Add more water if needed.

- Serve soup warm.

Nutrition

Calories: 187kcal

Fat: 12g

Phosphorus: 119mg

Potassium: 288mg

Sodium: 59mg

Carbohydrates: 7g

Protein: 11g

25. Green Bean Veggie Stew

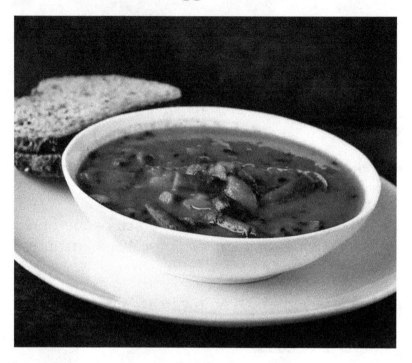

Preparation time: 10 minutes.

Cooking time: 35 minutes.

Servings: 2

Ingredients

- 6 cups shredded green cabbage
- 3 celery stalks, chopped
- 1 teaspoon unsalted butter
- ½ large sweet onion, chopped
- 1 teaspoon minced garlic

- 1 scallion, chopped

- 2 tablespoons chopped fresh parsley

- 2 tablespoons lemon juice

- 1 teaspoon chopped fresh oregano

- 1 tablespoon chopped fresh thyme

- 1 teaspoon chopped savory

- Water

- 1 cup fresh green beans, cut into 1-inch pieces

- Black pepper (ground), to taste

Directions

- Take a medium-large cooking pot, heat butter over medium heat.

- Add onion and stir-cook until become translucent and softened.

- Add garlic and stir-cook until you become fragrant.

- Add cabbage, celery, scallion, parsley, lemon juice, thyme, savory, and oregano; add water to cover veggies by 3–4 inches.

- Stir the mixture and boil it.

- Over low heat, cover, and simmer the mixture for about 25 minutes until veggies are tender.

- Add green beans and cook for 2–3 more minutes; season with black pepper to taste.

- Serve warm.

Nutrition

Calories: 56kcal

Fat: 1g

Phosphorus: 36mg

Potassium: 194mg

Sodium: 31mg

Carbohydrates: 7g

Protein: 1g

26. Chicken Pasta Soup

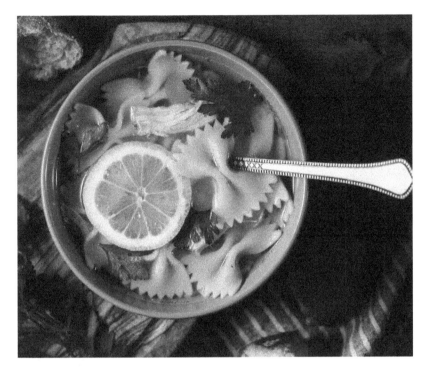

Preparation time: 10 minutes.

Cooking time: 20 minutes.

Servings: 6

Ingredients

- 1 ½ cups baby spinach

- 2 tablespoons orzo (tiny pasta)

- 1 tablespoon dry white wine

- 1 (14-ounce) low sodium chicken broth

- 2 plum tomatoes, chopped

- ½ teaspoon Italian seasoning

- 1 large shallot, chopped

- 1 small zucchini, diced

- 8-ounces chicken tenders

- 1 tablespoon extra-virgin olive oil

Directions

- Take a medium saucepan or skillet, add oil. Heat over medium heat.

- Add chicken and stir-cook for 3 minutes until evenly brown. Set aside.

- In the pan, add zucchini, Italian seasoning, shallot; stir-cook until veggies are softened.

- Add tomatoes, wine, broth, and orzo.

- Boil the mixture.

- Over low heat, cover, and simmer the mixture for about 3 minutes.

- Mix in spinach and cooked chicken; stir and serve warm.

Nutrition

Calories: 103kcal

Fat: 3g

Phosphorus: 125mg

Potassium: 264mg

Sodium: 84mg

Carbohydrates: 6g

Protein: 12g

27. Herbed Cabbage Stew

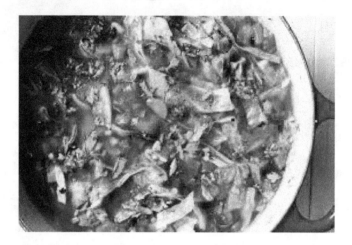

Preparation time: 20 minutes.

Cooking time: 35 minutes.

Servings: 2

Ingredients

- 1 teaspoon unsalted butter
- ½ large sweet onion, chopped
- 1 teaspoon minced garlic
- 6 cups shredded green cabbage
- 3 celery stalks, chopped with the leafy tops
- 1 scallion, both green and white parts, chopped
- 2 tablespoons chopped fresh parsley
- 2 tablespoons freshly squeezed lemon juice

- 1 tablespoon chopped fresh thyme

- 1 teaspoon chopped savory

- 1 teaspoon chopped fresh oregano

- Water

- Green beans, 1 cup, chopped

- Freshly ground black pepper

Directions

- In a medium stockpot over medium-high heat, melt the butter. Sauté the onion and garlic in the melted butter for about 3 minutes or until the vegetables are softened. Add the cabbage, celery, scallion, parsley, lemon juice, thyme, savory, and oregano to the pot, and add enough water to cover the vegetables by about 4 inches.

- Bring the soup to a boil, reduce the heat to low, and simmer the soup for about 25 minutes or until the vegetables are tender. Add the green beans and simmer 3 minutes; season with pepper.

Nutrition

Calories: 33kcal

Fat: 1g

Carbs: 6g

Phosphorus: 29mg

Potassium: 187mg

Sodium: 20mg

Protein: 1g

Vegetables and salads

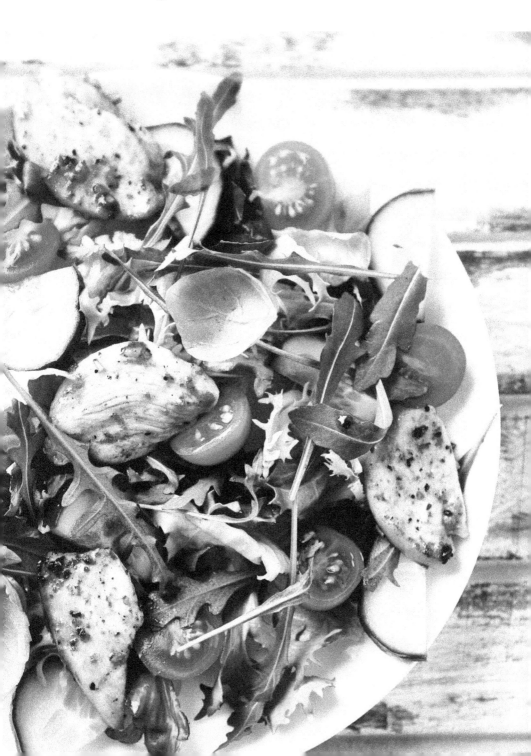

28. Cranberry Cabbage Slaw

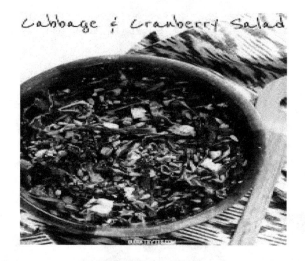

Cabbage & Cranberry Salad

Preparation time: 10 minutes.

Cooking time: 0 minutes.

Servings: 4

Ingredients

- 1/2 medium cabbage head, shredded

- 1 medium red apple, shredded

- 2 tablespoons onion, sliced

- 1/2 cup dried cranberries

- 1/4 cup almonds, toasted sliced

- 1/2 cup olive oil

- ¼ teaspoon stevia

- 1/4 cup cider vinegar

- 1/2 tablespoon celery seed

- 1/2 teaspoon dry mustard

- ½ cup cream

Directions

- Take a suitable salad bowl.

- Start tossing out all the ingredients.

- Mix well and serve.

Nutrition

Calories: 308kcal

Sodium: 23mg

Carbohydrate: 13.5g

Protein: 2.6g

Phosphorous: 257mg

Potassium: 219mg

29. Chestnut Noodle Salad

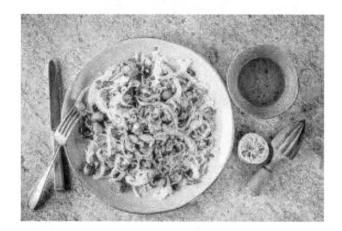

Preparation time: 10 minutes.

Cooking time: 0 minutes.

Servings: 6

Ingredients

- 8 cups cabbage, shredded
- 1/2 cup canned chestnuts, sliced
- 6 green onions, chopped
- 1/4 cup olive oil
- 1/4 cup apple cider vinegar
- 3/4 teaspoon stevia
- 1/8 teaspoon black pepper
- 1 cup chow Mein noodles, cooked

Directions

- Take a suitable salad bowl.

- Start tossing out all the ingredients.

- Mix well and serve.

Nutrition

Calories: 173kcal

Sodium: 78mg

Carbohydrate: 5.8g

Protein: 4.2g

Calcium: 142mg

Phosphorous: 188mg

Potassium: 302mg

30. Cranberry Broccoli Salad

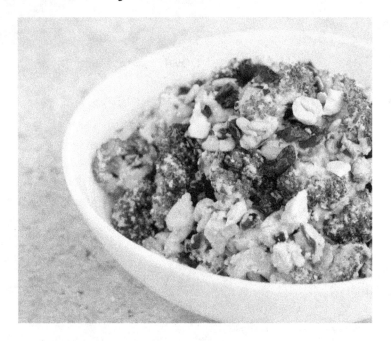

Preparation time: 10 minutes.

Cooking time: 0 minutes.

Servings: 4

Ingredients

- 3/4 cup plain Greek yogurt

- 1/4 cup mayonnaise

- 2 tablespoons maple syrup

- 2 tablespoons apple cider vinegar

- 4 cups broccoli florets

- 1 medium apple, chopped

- 1/2 cup red onion, sliced

- 1/4 cup parsley, chopped

- 1/2 cup dried cranberries

- 1/4 cup pecans

Directions

- Put all the salad ingredients into a suitable salad bowl.

- Toss them well and refrigerate for 1 hour.

- Serve.

Nutrition

Calories: 173kcal

Sodium: 157mg

Carbohydrate: 34g

Protein: 9.4g

Phosphorous: 291mg

Potassium: 480mg

31. Balsamic Beet Salad

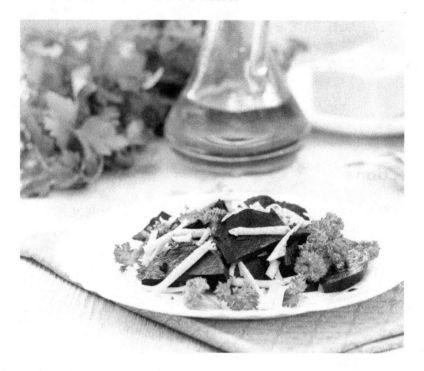

Preparation time: 10 minutes.

Cooking time: 0 minutes.

Servings: 2

Ingredients*:*

- 1 cucumber, peeled and sliced

- 15-ounces canned low-sodium beets, sliced

- 4 teaspoon balsamic vinegar

- 2 teaspoon sesame oil

- 2 tablespoons Gorgonzola cheese

Directions

- Take a suitable salad bowl.

- Start tossing in all the ingredients.

- Mix well and serve.

Nutrition:

Calories: 145kcal

Sodium: 426mg

Carbohydrate: 16.4g

Protein: 5g

Phosphorous: 79mg

Potassium: 229mg

32. Shrimp Salad

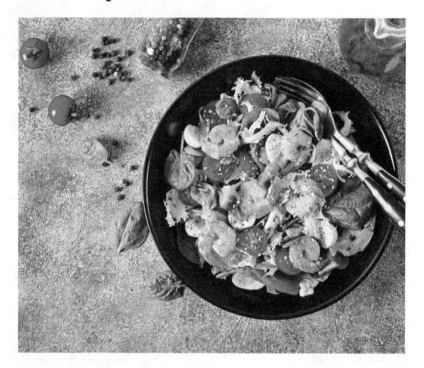

Preparation time: 10 minutes.

Cooking time: 0 minutes.

Servings: 4

Ingredients

- 1 pound shrimp, boiled and chopped
- 1 hardboiled egg, chopped
- 1 tablespoon celery, chopped
- 1 tablespoon green pepper, chopped
- 1 tablespoon onion, chopped

- 2 tablespoons mayonnaise
- 1 teaspoon lemon juice
- ½ teaspoon chili powder
- ⅛ teaspoon hot sauce
- ½ teaspoon dry mustard
- Lettuce, chopped or shredded

Directions

- Take a suitable salad bowl.
- Start tossing in all the ingredients.
- Mix well and serve.

Nutrition

Calories: 173kcal

Sodium: 381mg

Carbohydrate: 4.3g

Protein: 27.5g

Phosphorous: 249mg

Potassium: 233mg

Drink and Smoothies

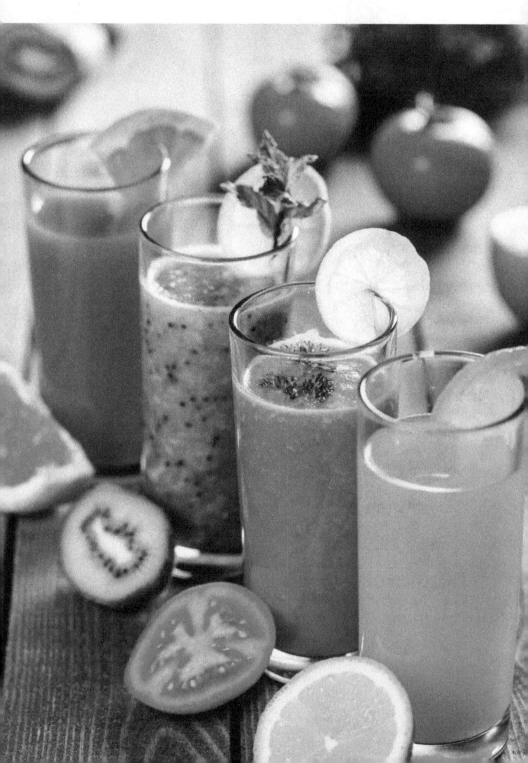

33. Collard Greens and Cucumber Smoothie

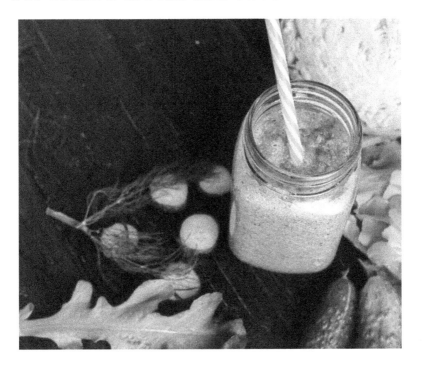

Preparation time: 15 minutes.

Cooking time: 0 minute.

Servings: 2

Ingredients

- 1 cup collard greens
- A few fresh peppermints leaves
- 1 big cucumber
- 1 lime, freshly juiced
- 1/2 cups avocado sliced

- 1 1/2 cup water

- 1 cup crushed ice

- 1/4 cup natural sweetener Erythritol or Stevia (optional)

Directions

- Rinse and clean your collard greens from any dirt.

- Place all ingredients in a food processor or blender,

- Blend until all ingredients in your smoothie are combined well.

- Pour in a glass and drink. Enjoy!

Nutrition

Calories: 123kcal

Carbohydrates: 8g

Proteins: 4g

Fat: 11g

Fiber: 6g

34. Creamy Dandelion Greens and Celery Smoothie

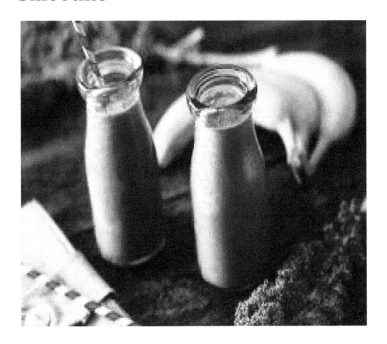

Preparation time: 10 minutes.

Cooking time: 0 minute.

Servings: 2

Ingredients

- 1 handful raw dandelion greens

- 2 celery sticks

- 2 tablespoon chia seeds

- 1 small piece of ginger, minced

- 1/2 cup almond milk

- 1/2 cup of water

- 1/2 cup plain yogurt

Directions:

- Rinse and clean dandelion leaves from any dirt; add in a high-speed blender.

- Clean the ginger; keep only the inner part and cut into small slices; add in a blender.

- Add all remaining ingredients and blend until smooth.

- Serve and enjoy!

Nutrition

Calories: 58kcal

Carbohydrates: 5g

Proteins: 3g

Fat: 6g

Fiber: 3g

35. Dark Turnip Greens Smoothie

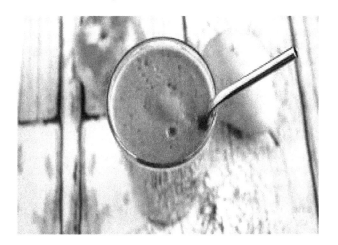

Preparation time: 10 minutes.

Cooking time: 0 minute.

Servings: 2

Ingredients

- 1 cup raw turnip greens

- 1 1/2 cup almond milk

- 1 tablespoon almond butter

- 1/2 cup water

- 1/2 teaspoon cocoa powder, unsweetened

- 1 tablespoon dark chocolate chips

- 1/4 teaspoon cinnamon

- A pinch salt

- 1/2 cup crushed ice

Directions

- Rinse and clean turnip greens from any dirt.

- Place the turnip greens in your blender along with all other ingredients.

- Blend it for 45–60 seconds or until done; smooth and creamy.

- Serve with or without crushed ice.

Nutrition

Calories: 131kcal

Carbohydrates: 6g

Proteins: 4g

Fat: 10g

Fiber: 2.5g

36. Butter Pecan and Coconut Smoothie

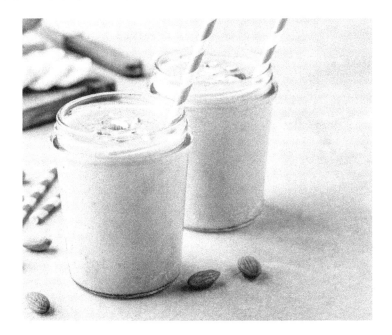

Preparation time: 10 minutes.

Cooking time: 0 minute.

Servings: 2

Ingredients

- 1 cup coconut milk, canned
- 1 scoop butter pecan powdered creamer
- 2 cups fresh spinach leaves, chopped
- 1/2 banana frozen or fresh
- 2 tablespoon stevia granulated sweetener to taste
- 1/2 cup water

- 1 cup ice cubes crushed

Directions

- Place ingredients from the list above in your high-speed blender.

- Blend for 35–50 seconds or until all ingredients combined well.

- Add less or more crushed ice.

- Drink and enjoy!

Nutrition

Calories: 268kcal

Carbohydrates: 7g

Proteins: 6g

Fat: 26g

Fiber: 1.5g

37. Fresh Cucumber, Kale, and Raspberry Smoothie

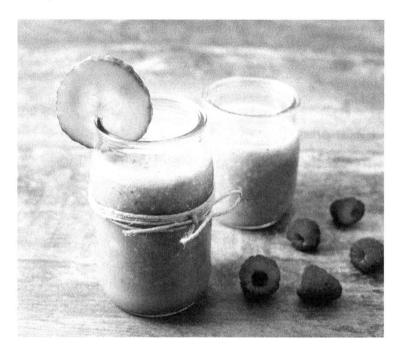

Preparation time: 10 minutes.

Cooking time: 0 minute.

Servings: 3

Ingredients

- 1 1/2 cups cucumber, peeled

- 1/2 cup raw kale leaves

- 1 1/2 cups fresh raspberries

- 1 cup almond milk

- 1 cup water

- Ice cubes crushed (optional)

- 2 tablespoons natural sweetener (Stevia, Erythritol, etc.)

Directions

- Place all ingredients from the list in a food processor or high-speed blender and blend for 35–40 seconds.

- Serve into chilled glasses.

- Add more natural sweeter if you like. Enjoy!

Nutrition

Calories: 70kcal

Carbohydrates: 8g

Proteins: 3g

Fat: 6g

Fiber: 5g

38. Protein Coconut Smoothie

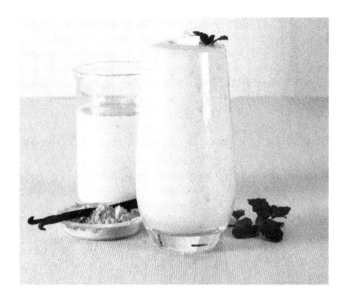

Preparation time: 10 minutes.

Cooking time: 0 minutes.

Servings: 2

Ingredients

- 1 1/2 cup coconut milk canned

- 1 cup fresh spinach finely chopped

- 1 scoop vanilla protein powder

- 2 tablespoons chia seeds

- 1 cup ice cubes crushed

- 2–3 tablespoons stevia granulated natural sweetener (optional)

Directions

- Rinse and clean your spinach leaves from any dirt.

- Place all ingredients from the list above in a blender.

- Blend until you get a smoothie, like always.

- Serve in a cold glass and it is ready to drink.

Nutrition

Calories: 377kcal

Carbohydrates: 7g

Proteins: 10g

Fat: 38g

Fiber: 2g

Dessert

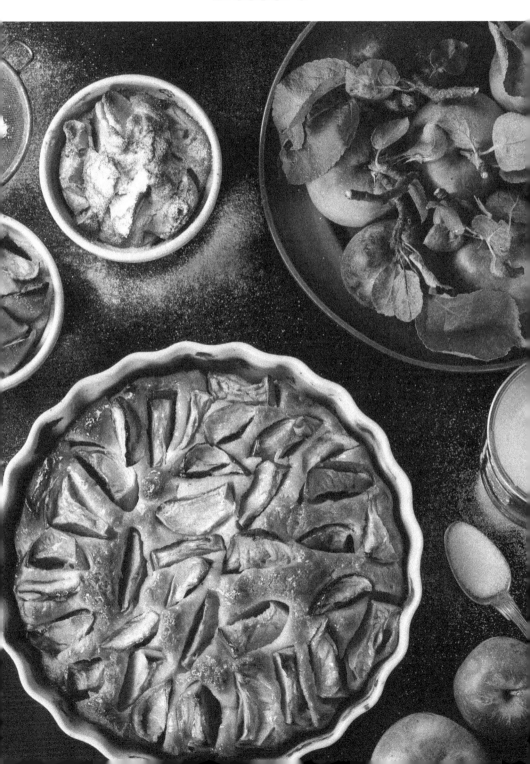

39. Strawberry Whipped Cream Cake

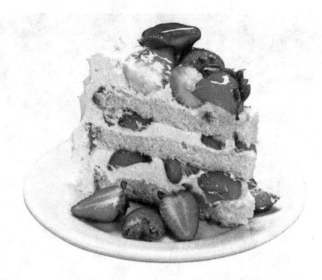

Preparation time: 10 minutes.

Cooking time: 30 minutes.

Servings: 4

Ingredients

- 1-pint whipping cream

- 2 tablespoon gelatin

- 1/2 glass cold water

- 1 glass boiling water

- 3 tablespoon lemon juice

- 1 orange glass juice

- 1 orange glass juice

- 1 teaspoon sugar

- 3/4 cup sliced strawberries

- 1 large angel food cake or light sponge cake

Direction

- Put the gelatin in cold water, then add hot water and blend. Add orange and lemon juice, also add some sugar and go on blending.

- Refrigerate and leave it there until you see it is starting to gel.

- Whip half portion of cream, add it to the mixture along with strawberries, put wax paper in the bowl and cut the cake into small pieces.

- In between the pieces, add the whipped cream and put everything in the fridge for one night.

- When you take out the cake, add some whipped cream on top and decorate with some more fruit. Serve and enjoy!

Nutrition

Calories: 355kcal

Protein: 4g

Sodium: 275mg

Potassium: 145mg

Phosphorus: 145mg

40. Sweet Cracker Pie Crust

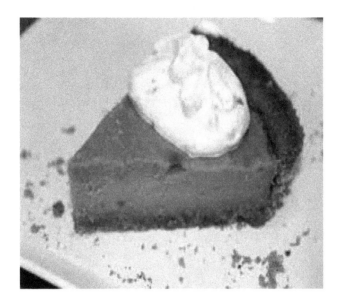

Preparation time: 10 minutes.

Cooking time: 7 minutes.

Servings: 2

Ingredients

- 1 bowl gelatin cracker crumbs

- 1/4 small cup sugar

- Unsalted butter

Direction

- Mix sweet cracker crumbs, butter and sugar.

- Heat the oven to 375°F.

- Bake for 7 minutes, putting it in a greased pie.

- Let the pie cool before adding any kind of filling. Serve and enjoy!

Nutrition

Calories: 205kcal

Protein: 2g

Sodium: 208mg

Potassium: 67mg

Phosphorus: 22mg

41. Apple Oatmeal Crunchy

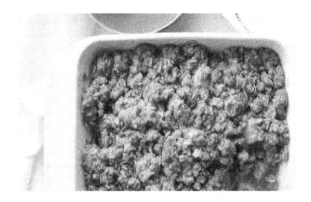

Preparation time: 10 minutes.

Cooking time: 40 minutes.

Servings: 2

Ingredients

- 5 green apples
- 1 bowl oatmeal
- A small cup brown sugar
- 1/2 cup flour
- 1 teaspoon cinnamon
- 1/2 bowl butter

Direction

- Prepare apples by cutting them into tiny slices and preheat the oven at 350°F.

- In a cup mix oatmeal, flour, cinnamon and brown sugar.

- Put butter in the batter and place sliced apple in a baking pan (9" x 13").

- Spread the oatmeal mixture over the apples and bake for 35 minutes. Serve and enjoy!

Nutrition

Calories: 295kcal

Protein: 3g

Sodium: 95mg

Potassium: 190mg

Phosphorus: 73mg

42. Berry Ice Cream

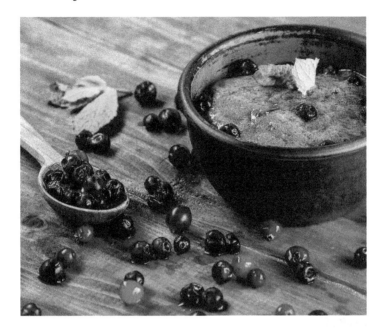

Preparation time: 10 minutes.

Cooking time: 60 minutes.

Servings: 2

Ingredients

- 6 ice cream cones
- 1 cup whipped topping
- 1 cup fresh blueberries
- 4 ounces cream cheese
- 1/4 cup blueberry jam

Direction

- Put the cream cheese in a large cup and beat it with a mixer until it is fluffy.

- Mix with fruit and jam and whipped topping.

- Put the mixture on the small ice cream cones and refrigerate them in the freezer for 1 hour or more until they are ready to serve. Enjoy!

Nutrition

Calories: 175kcal

Protein: 3g

Sodium: 95mg

Potassium: 80mg

Phosphorus: 40mg

Conclusion

Following a Renal Diet means following a diet that may be less taxing on your kidneys and, therefore, may slow the development of kidney disease. Kidney disease is a serious health problem that you can take sitting down.

Not only should you follow a healthy kidney-friendly diet if you are at risk of or have already been diagnosed with kidney problems; you should also manage other medical conditions that can affect the kidneys, as well as maintain an ideal weight.

You should also make sure that these practices become a habit for you and you will definitely start to notice a positive change in your overall health.

CPSIA information can be obtained
at www.ICGtesting.com
Printed in the USA
BVHW062014190321
602997BV00005B/256